THE ESSENTIAL KETO DIET BOOK FOR WOMEN

Lose Weight with Quick and Healthy Recipes for Everyday incl. 21 Days Diet Plan

[1st Edition]

Weight Loss Experts

TABLE OF CONTENTS

« Keto » Diet and Helpful Tips

« Keto » Explained

Keto diet is a perfect solution for you if you want to lose weight, yet still be healthy and enjoy your favorite food. It is trendy and combines elements of international cuisine and fusion kitchen. You are also free to experiment if you have allergies or avoid certain foods. This book combines a variety of delicious recipes that can satisfy even the most picky gourmets and cooks with different personal references, and I am sure you will be able to find something that is up to your taste.

Keto diet is relatively new phenomenon in the dietary world. However, we all have heard dieticians and health specialist about balancing your diet with fruits and veggies.

Most dieticians' advice to eat less meat, carbohydrates, but caution not to fall into a trap of exhausting your body by sitting on a diet for too long. That may cause anorexique disorder or bulimia and you may end up in a hospital instead of a healthy body that one hoped to achieve from a diet.

What is « Keto » Diet?

Keto diet is a low carb diet that is similar to low fat diets and veganism, yet more balanced and healthy as it still involves meat products and foods that have natural fat. Keto diet is somewhat similar to Atkins diet. It is perfect for people who are lactose intolerant and have an allergic reaction to gluten as the emphasis is made on cutting carbohydrates.

Getting Ready

To get ready for a diet is a complex procedure. You must be physically, spiritually and mentally prepared to cut off some of the habits, foods and strengthen your spirit to be able to keep in promises to follow through with the dietary course and hit the target that you have to set for yourself. That way it will be easier for you to stay motivated and focused on a desired goal.

You have to be spiritually ready to work on your body and achieve the dream size. In order to be satisfied within, you have to love your body, otherwise you will like diet is a torture and no results will be achieved: after diet, the gained weight will come back at even faster rate as it was lost. First of all, Keto Diet is a lifestyle and it is easy to make it fun and enjoyable experience.

Losing Weight Effectively

In order to lose weight effectively and not just for a few days, you have to set up your kitchen wisely, so you do not have a temptation to come back to the previous lifestyle. Healthy eating **requires effort** and you have to make that extra step to achieve your dream body and keep the result for long time.

Useful Tips

Set up kitchen and fridge. Clear kitchen of unhealthy food that would distract you from staying on track. Finish all the food that is full of carbohydrates or give it to your neighbors. You must not have a temptation of going back to starch and carbs.

No dining in bed. Make sure that your lifestyle is corresponding with your diet. « Lasy » week-end in bad may throw you back into dining full of « bad » saturated fats and carbs.

Clear space for new products, thoughts, places. Keto diet involves not only food aspect, but also combination of it with healthy lifestyle: do sports, go for a walk, do yoga or gym. That will ensure you a better result.

Make a list of products that includes more fruits than vegetable.

Keep the diary to cheer yourself and be on track. Records will help you to stay closer to a desired number target on a scale.

Treat yourself for every goal that achieved. Keto diet has many healthy treat options, so you can treat yourself with a tasty sweet once you get close to your target. Set small goals, so it is easier to be on track and avoid abrupt and harsh response of your body.

Supporting Material

Please, consult with your physician if you are not sure whether Keto Diet is a good option for you or if you have allergies to certain products or other concerns. They may provide you with a guideline or refer to dietician.

PART 2: RECIPES

Breakfast

Breakfast is one of the most important meals of the day in Keto diet. Please, never skip it even if « do not feel like it ». The regular food intake sets your body in a right order to function « like a clock », so each meal is not heavy on your stomach and to avoid overeating at nighttime.

Classic Scrambled Eggs with Bacon

Ready in 8 minutes | Serves 2 people | 544 calories

Ingredients:

- 2 tsp. butter
- 4 large eggs
- 2 tbsp of heavy cream
- Pinch of salt, to taste
- Ground pepper
- 4 slices bacon

Preparation:

1. In large bowl, beat the eggs with cream salt and pepper;
2. Whip vigorously for few minutes until eggs are evenly colored and slightly froth.
3. Do not overbeat eggs.
4. Melt butter in skillet over medium heat.
5. Once butter is melted, pour in the egg mixture and cook it for 1 minute.
6. Push spatula through to the opposite edge, allowing uncooked egg to redistribute.
7. Continue this process until egg mixture is no longer runny.
8. Season eggs with salt and pepper to taste and transfer to a serving plate.
9. To cook bacon, place a skillet over high heat. No need to use oil or butter because of the high fat content of the bacon.
10. Lay strips of bacon in the skillet next to each other without overlapping. Bacon will start sizzling and popping as the skillet heats up.
11. Allow bakon to cook until it starts to wrinkle and forms waves. It should not stick to the bottom of the skillet. Use fork or tongs to turn bacon over and cook for 2 to 3 minutes.

12. Keep frying bacon until it is crisp, red-brown in color, and no longer shows any white or pink areas.

13. Transfer to a plate with eggs and serve warm.

Tips

Use paper towels to absorb extra fat from bacon.

Cauliflower Fritters

Ready in 20 minutes | Serves 2 people | 920 calories

Ingredients:

- 1 lb cauliflower florets
- 1 cup shredded cheddar cheese
- 2 large eggs
- 2 tbsp coconut flour
- 2 tbsp finely chopped scallions
- 1 tbsp of sour cream
- 2 tbsp of olive oil
- Salt
- Pepper

Preparation:

1. Shred the cauliflower with a food processor or grater.
2. Steam cauliflower until tender.
3. Mix in cheese with cauliflower while the cauliflower is still hot, until cheese is melted and evenly mixed in.
4. Add in eggs, coconut flour and scallions.
5. Mix until everything is evenly combined.
6. Preheat skillet and once you hear oil popping, it is ready to fry pancakes.
7. Make little balls out of mixture and fry until golden. Press gently with a fork to make pancake shape.
8. Serve hot with sour cream.

Tips

Be careful not to overcook cauliflower. It may become mushy if you cook it for more than 5 minutes.

Avocado Stuffed Eggs

Ready in 40 minutes | Serves 2 people | 254 calories

Ingredients:

- 2 slices bacon, diced
- 6 large eggs
- 1 avocado, halved, seeded and peeled
- 2 tablespoons chopped fresh cilantro leaves
- 1 tablespoon freshly squeezed lemon juice
- Zest of 1 lemon
- Kosher salt and freshly ground black pepper, to taste
- 2 tablespoons chopped fresh chives
- 1 jalapeno pepper

Preparation:

1. Place eggs in a large pot and bring to a boil and cook for 6 minutes.
2. Remove from heat and place eggs into cold water for 8-10 minutes. That will make the eggs easier to peel.
3. Cut the eggs in half lengthwise, reserving the yolks.
4. In a small bowl, mash the yolks and avocado with a fork until chunky.
5. Stir in cilantro, lemon juice and lemon zest; season with salt and pepper, to taste.
6. Use a pastry bag or ziplock bag with a corner thinly cut fitted with to pipe into the eggs,
7. Heat a large skillet over medium high heat. Add bacon and cook until brown and crispy, about 6-8 minutes.
8. Transfer to a paper towel-lined plate; set aside.
9. Top your eggs with bacon and garnish with chives and jalapeno pepper, for zesty flavor.

Tips

Prepare it ahead of time for a tasty breakfast. You may store it in a fridge for up to 3 hours.

French Omelette

Ready in 7 minutes | Serves 1 serving | 178 calories

Ingredients:

- 2 large eggs
- Pinch of salt
- Dash of ground pepper to taste
- 1 tsp. of unsalted butter
- 1/3 cup filling, such as shredded cheese

Preparation:

1. Beat eggs vigorously until foam is formed, add salt and pepper in small bowl until blended.
2. Melt butter in 6 to 8-inch nonstick omelet pan over medium-high heat until hot.
3. Pour egg mixture into pan. Mixture should set immediately at edges.
4. The French omelette should be smooth, unbrowned,
5. Cook slowly over medium-low to medium heat, with initial stirring to prevent curds and sticking.
6. When top surface of eggs is thickened and no visible liquid egg remains,
7. Put filling on one side of the omelet.
8. Fold omelet in half with turner. With a quick flip of the wrist, turn pan and slide omelette onto plate.

Tips

Serve immediately.

Mexican Style Omelette

Ready in 15minutes | Serves 1 serving | 191 calories

Ingredients:

- 4 medium eggs
- 2 teaspoons olive oil
- 1 small jalapeno, thinly sliced and seeded, stem discarded
- 1/2 cup diced red onion
- 1 clove garlic, minced
- handful of grape or cherry tomatoes, halved

Preparation:

1. Just saute up your filling Ingredients: in a skillet.
2. Transfer them to a separate plate, and cook your egg whites into a big pancake.
3. Add your filling Ingredients: back in at the end, then fold it over, and sprinkle with some extra cheese and cilantro on top for garnish..

Tips

Serve hot for cheese to be chewy.

Breakfast Quesadillas

Ready in 20 minutes | Serves 2 people | 695 calories

Ingredients:

- 1 Chicken Breast
- 1 Onion
- 30 grams of grated cheddar cheese
- 1 Bell Pepper
- 2 Flour Tortillas
- Dash of Tex-Mex Spices
- Sour cream

Preparation:

1. Preheat grill and spray it with olive oil
2. Marinade chicken breast for 5 minutes. Add sliced chicken, onions and bell pepper together with spices.
3. Cook for 10 minutes. Make sure it is cooked throughout.
4. Remove from the grill.
5. Prepare tortillas: put one tortilla on the grill to be the bottom of fajita. Put cooked chicken mixture together with cheddar cheese and cover it with another tortilla.
6. Grill for 3 minutes. Then turn and cook for another couple of minutes.
7. Remove from grill
8. Cut into 8 even slices.
9. Serve hot with sour cream.

Tips

You may also try serving it with guacamole or salsa.

Apple Pancakes

Ready in 20 minutes | Serves 2 people | 600 calorie

Ingredients:

- 🍽 Large green apple
- 🍽 2 large eggs
- 🍽 ¼ milk
- 🍽 2 tbsp olive oil
- 🍽 4 tbsp. of flour
- 🍽 1 tsp of baking soda
- 🍽 ½ tsp of cinnamon

Preparation:

1. Heat up oil in a large skillet until very hot.
2. Peel apple and grate it.
3. Add eggs, milk, cinnamon, flour and baking powder
4. Mix carefully all the Ingredients:.
5. Make pancakes and fry until golden brown.
6. Serve hot.

Tips

Serve with agave syrup or low-calorie apple jelly.

Banana Pancakes

Ready in 20 minutes | Serves 2 people | 600 calories

Ingredients:

- 2 large ripe bananas with spots
- 2 tsp of baking soda
- 1 tsp vanilla extract
- 2 large eggs
- 4-6 Tbsp coconut or almond flour

Preparation:

1. Heat up oil in a large skillet until very hot.
2. Peel banana and mash it with a fork.
3. Add eggs, flour, baking powder and vanilla extract.
4. Mix all the Ingredients: together.
5. Make pancakes and fry until golden brown.
6. Serve hot.

Tips

Serve with agave syrup or melted peanut butter.

Banana Waffles with Vanilla Custard

Ready in 50 minutes | Serves 4 people | 1030 calories or 257 calories per serving

Ingredients:

For Custard:

- 1 vanilla pod
- 2 ½ cup of 2% milk
- 4 large free-range egg yolks
- 2 tablespoons caster sugar
- 1 tablespoon cornflour

Pancakes:

- 1 1/4 cups all-purpose flour
- 3 tsp of baking powder
- 1/2 tsp of salt
- 1 pinch ground nutmeg
- 1 cup 1% milk
- 1 egg
- 2 ripe bananas, mashed

Preparation:

For Custard:

1. Halve the vanilla pod and scrape out the seeds. Add both the pod and seeds to a pan on a medium-low heat, pour in the milk and bring just to the boil.
2. Remove from the heat and leave to cool slightly, then pick out the vanilla pod.
3. In a large mixing bowl, whisk the egg yolks with the sugar and cornflour until pale.
4. Gradually add the warm milk, a small amount at a time, whisking well before each addition.
5. Pour the mixture back into the pan and cook gently on a low heat for about 20 minutes or until thickened, whisking continuously. Delicious served with all kinds of crumble

While Custard is cooking, start making pancakes.

1. Preheat waffle iron.
2. In a large mixing bowl put bananas, sift together flour, baking powder, salt and nutmeg.
3. Stir in milk and eggs until mixture is smooth.
4. Spray preheated waffle iron with non-stick cooking spray.
5. Pour 4 tbsp of the banana batter onto the hot waffle iron.
6. Cook until golden brown.
7. Serve hot with vanilla custard on top.

Tips

Cook on low heat and do not panic if eggs will start to stick to the pan. Simply remove it from heat and let it cool. Then place it back on low heat.

Fruit Salad

Ready in 5 minutes | Serves 1 serving | 150 calories

Ingredients:

- 1 slice of melon
- 1 slice of watermelon
- Few grapes
- 1 Kiwi
- 2 Strawberries
- Blueberries
- 1 pineapple ring

Preparation:

1. Chop all the Ingredients: into cubes, except grapes
2. Mix well and enjoy!

Tips

You may add Greek yogurt as sauce.

Oatmeal Cereal with Chocolate Chips

Ready in 5 minutes | Serves 1 serving | 150 calories

Ingredients:

- 1 cup of oatmeal cereal
- ¼ cup of 70 % cocoa chocolate chips
- 1 small banana
- 1 cup of milk or hot water

Preparation:

1. Preheat small pot.
2. Pour milk and let it simmer 2 minutes.
3. Add cereal.
4. Boil cereal for 2-3 minutes.
5. Remove from heat.
6. Serve in a bowl and add chocolate chips and a sliced banana.

Tips

Serve hot.

Does not require additional sweeteners.

Oatmeal Cereal with Berry Mix

Ready in 5minutes | Serves 1 serving | 150 calories

Ingredients:

- 🍽 1 cup of oatmeal cereal
- 🍽 1 cup of water
- 🍽 ¼ cup of Blueberries
- 🍽 ¼ of Strawberries
- 🍽 1 tbsp of crushed walnuts
- 🍽 1 tbsp of pumpkin seeds
- 🍽 1 tsp of flax seeds

Preparation:

1. Preheat small pot.
2. Pour water and let it simmer 2 minutes.
3. Add cereal.
4. Boil cereal for 2-3 minutes.
5. Remove from heat.
6. Serve in a bowl and add berry mix and seeds.

Tips

You may make it sweeter by adding agave syrup or sweeteners.

Oatmeal Cereal with Coconut

Ready in 5 minutes | Serves 1 serving | 150 calories

Ingredients:

- 1 cup of oatmeal cereal
- 1 cup of milk
- 1 tbsp of brown sugar
- 2 tbsp of coconut flakes

Preparation:

1. Preheat small pot.
2. Pour milk and let it simmer 2 minutes.
3. Add cereal.
4. Boil cereal for 2-3 minutes.
5. Remove from heat.
6. Serve in a bowl and add coconut flakes and brown sugar.

Tips

You may replace brown sugar by agave syrup and instead of coconut add apples and cinnamon.

Egg Sandwich with Avocado

Ready in 10 minutes | Serves 1 serving | 460 calories

Ingredients:

- 🍽 2 large eggs
- 🍽 1 ripe avocado
- 🍽 2 slices of whole wheat bread

Preparation:

1. Boil eggs for 5 minutes
2. Place eggs for 5 minutes into cold water to cool and it will make it easier to peel them from the shell.
3. Peel avocado and mash it with a fork.
4. Peel eggs and slice them into thin halfs or ovals.
5. Toast bread slices.
6. Spread avocado on toasts and put egg rings.

Tips

If the eggs are fresh it will be hard to peel them. Place them into a cold water for longer and change it if necessary. That should help to separate eggs from shells. Make sure they are 1-2 day old.

Check whether avocado is ripe. Green fresh avocados are hard to mash. Ripe avocado should have darker skin.

Egg White Wrap with Feta Cheese and Spinach

Ready in 20 minutes | Serves 1 serving | 280 calories

Ingredients:

- 2 Egg whites
- 1 tbsp of olive oil
- ½ cup spinach
- 20 grams of feta cheese (or salted cottage cheese)
- 1 flour tortilla

Preparation:

1. Separate egg writes and beat them well
2. Preheat skilled and pour olive oil.
3. Fry egg whites for 3 minutes or until just ready, do not let it get a golden color.
4. In the same pan simmer spinach for 5 minutes
5. Place cottage cheese, spinach and fried egg white on tortilla.
6. Wrap well in an envelope style.
7. Grill for 2-3 minutes.

Tips

Do not overlook egg whites, if the skillet is hot sometimes 1 minute is enough.

Zucchini Hash Browns

Ready in 20 minutes | Serves 4 people | 143 calories per serving

Ingredients:

- 2 medium zucchinis
- 1/2 onion
- salt to taste
- 1/2 cup of grated parmesan
- 1/3 cup chives
- 2 tbsp of olive oil

Preparation:

1. Preheat skillet to 400 degrees F. Pour olive oil.
2. Use a box grater to coarsely grate the zucchini and onion.
3. Place grated zucchini and onion into a large mixing bowl. Sprinkle with salt, mix, and statin form an excess liquid.
4. Place the strained zucchini mixture back into the large bowl and add remaining Ingredients:. Mix until well combined.
5. Form patties out of the mixture and place on a pan for about 7-8 minutes, until underside is golden and crispy. Flip hash brown patties and continue to cook for an additional 5 minutes.
6. Serve warm.

Tips

The salt will draw moisture out of the zucchini. Strain the excess moisture out of the zucchini by placing the zucchini mixture into a kitchen towel and twisting tightly.

If you want to cut on a few calories, you may also bake hash browns.

Eggs Benedict with Salmon

Ready in 30 minutes | Serves 1 serving | 759 calories

Ingredients:

- 2 medium eggs
- 50 grams of smoked salmon
- 2 slices of whole wheat bread
- 1 tbsp of vinegar for cooking
- 1 tbsp of capers
- ½ cup of Seasonal greens, spinach

For Sauce:

- 3 egg yolks
- ¼ cup of water
- 2 tbsp of lemon juice
- ½ butter (cut into 8 pieces)
- 1/4 tsp. salt,
- 1/8 tsp. paprika and
- dash of ground pepper

Preparation:

1. To poach an egg, first fill the pot with about 3 inches of water. Bring the water to a boil and then reduce heat until it reaches a simmer. Add a little splash of vinegar to the water (this is optional, but it helps the egg white to stay together once it is in the water).
2. Crack one egg into a small cup or use a measuring cup. Lower the egg into the simmering water, gently easing it out of the cup.
3. Cook the egg in on low heat for 3-5 minutes, depending on how soft you want your egg yolk. Remove the poached egg with a spoon.
4. Toast your bread.
5. Place salmon with capers, greens, poached egg on toast and cover it with Béchamel sauce.

Sauce Béchamel

1. Whisk egg yolks, 1/4 cup water and 2 tbsp. fresh lemon juice in small saucepan until blended.
2. Cook over very low heat, stirring constantly, until mixture bubbles at the edges.
3. Stir in butter, one piece at a time, until butter is melted and until sauce is thickened.
4. Remove from heat.
5. Stir in spices.
6. It should make about ¾ of a cup of sauce. Serve warm.

Tips

Cool sauce on a low heat. Remove from the stove if necessary, let it cool off and then continue cooking on lower heat.

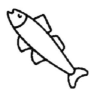

Egg Salad

Ready in 20 minutes | Serves 1 serving | 400 calories

Ingredients:

- 4 large eggs
- ¼ cup of chives
- ½ light mayonnaise
- Whole grain crackers
- Salt to taste
- Dash of ground pepper

Preparation:

1. Boil eggs until hard for 6 minutes
2. Peel and dice into cubes
3. Add sliced chives, mayonnaise, salt and pepper to taste.
4. Serve with whole wheat crackers.

Tips

Best served with whole grain crackers.

Snacks

Snacks are very important part your diet. Do not exhaust your body by starvation, better take small amounts of food more frequently, than large portions once or twice a day. That will make your stomach heavy and bad for your digestion. Make snacks a habit. Take at least two snacks a day - in the morning before lunch and in the afternoon before supper. That will satisfy your craving for food and will make you feel full before the actual meal. Some snacks can be full meal replacements and quite nutritious, so if your snack was full of calories and you don't feel that hungry - make a lighter lunch or dinner. Also, watch your calorie intake, make sure that your snack is light and do not abuse nutrition bars, - they will make you gain weight, rather than lose it. Nutrition bars were designed so you don't starve and to make a quick snack in between main course meals, not to replace it.

Blueberry Smoothie

Ready in 5 minutes | Serves 2 servings | 250 calories

Ingredients:

- 1/2 cup nonfat or 1 % milk
- 1/2 cup non-fat plain yogurt
- 1 cup frozen blueberries
- 1 teaspoon honey

Preparation:

1. Mix in blender until smooth.

Tips

May add another type of syrup like agave nectar to replace honey.

Raspberry Smoothie

Ready in 5 minutes | Serves 2 servings | 300 calories

Ingredients:

- 1/2 cup nonfat or 1 % milk
- 1/2 cup non-fat plain yogurt
- 1 cup frozen raspberries
- 1 cup of frozen peaches
- 2 tbsp of fresh lemon juice
- 1 teaspoon honey

Preparation:

1. Mix in blender until smooth.

Tips

Boost your smoothie by adding flaxseed, chia seeds, protein powder, wheat germ, or anything else that might give your smoothie a higher nutritional value.

Pomegranate Smoothie

Ready in 5 minutes | Serves 2 servings | 300 calories

Ingredients:

- ½ cup nonfat or 1 % milk
- 1/2 cup non-fat plain yogurt
- 1 cup of pomegranate seeds
- 1/2 cup of frozen raspberries
- ½ cup of blueberries or black currants
- ½ cup of blackberries
- 1 teaspoon honey

Preparation:

1. Mix in a blender or magic bullet until smooth.
2. Add kale or other seeds like chia seeds to increase nutritional value (optional).

Ginger Smoothie

Ready in 5 minutes | Serves 2 servings | 400 calories

Ingredients:

- 1/2 cup frozen peaches
- 1/2 cup frozen pineapple
- 1/2 cup frozen mango
- juice of 1 whole, large lemon
- 1/2 tbsp of lemon zest
- 3/4 cup unsweetened coconut milk
- 1 tbsp of freshly grated ginger
- 1/2 tbsp of honey
- 2 tbsp protein powder of choice
- 1 tbsp of chia seeds

Preparation:

1. Mix all the ingredients in a blender on a high speed until smooth.

Tips

Add boost with your favorite protein shake.

Mango Smoothie

Ready in 5 minutes | Serves 2 servings | 400 calories

Ingredients:

- fresh mangoes or 2 cups of frozen mango
- 1 frozen banana, can use unfrozen if using frozen mango
- 1/2 cup of almond milk

Preparation:

1. Mix in a blender for 1 minute on high speed until smooth.

Tips

Add your favorite protein boost, optional.

Celery Pineapple Smoothie

Ready in 5minutes | Serves 2 servings | 400 calories

Ingredients:

- 1 banana
- 3 stalks of celery
- 1 pear
- 1 cup of pineapple
- 1/2 cup of almond milk, unsweetened

Preparation:

1. Mix well in a blender until smooth.

Chia Pudding

Ready in 20 minutes | Serves 8 people | 280 calories

Ingredients:

- 1 cup of coconut or almond milk
- 2 tbsp of chia seeds
- vanilla stevia drops or other sweetener
- optional fruit and granola toppings of choice

Preparation:

1. In a cup put chia seeds and pour milk over.
2. Let it sit in a fridge for 20 minutes
3. Add sweetener and decorate with fruits or add granola, nuts or other toppings.

Tips

Add your favorite seeds and nuts to boost nutritional value.

Banana Chocolate Smoothie

Ready in 5 minutes | Serves 1 serving | 400 calories

Ingredients:

- 🍽 1 banana
- 🍽 ½ cup of protein boost
- 🍽 ½ cup of plain yogurt
- 🍽 ¼ of cocoa powder
- 🍽 1 cup of almond milk, unsweetened

Preparation:

1. Mix well in a blender on high speed until smooth for 1 minute

Strawberry Smoothie

Ready in 2 minutes | Serves 1 serving | 350 calories

Ingredients:

- 1 banana
- 2 cups of diced strawberries (about 6)
- ½ cup of plain yogurt
- 1 cup of pineapple
- 1/2 cup of almond milk, unsweetened

Preparation:

1. Mix well in a blender until smooth.
2. Add oatmeal or flax seeds for boost (optional)

Lunch

Lunch is one of the main dining of the day. It is a half day meal course when your body is the most active and burns most calories. Make it nutritious, fuel your body with healthy and full of vitamins product. Make sure there is enough protein and vegetables on your plate.

Light Chicken Cutlets

Ready in 20 minutes | Serves 5 servings or cutlets | 635 calories

Ingredients:

- 1 pound of minced chicken
- 1 onion
- 2 eggs
- 2 tbsp of flour
- 2 tbsp of olive oil
- Salt to taste
- Dash of ground pepper

Preparation:

1. Preheat skillet and pour oil on it.
2. Chop onions
3. Mix all the Ingredients: carefully , except flour, add salt and pepper.
4. Form Cutlets, a size of about 2 inches.
5. Fry until golden brown.

Tips

Serve with lemon and steamed vegetables on the side.

Butternut Squash Salad

Ready in 40 minutes | Serves 1 serving | 450 calories

Ingredients:

- 1 cup bulgur
- 2 cups water
- 1 small butternut squash (about 1 and 1/2 pounds)
- 2 1/2 tbsp olive oil, divided
- pinch of salt
- 1/3 cup of pumpkin seeds
- 6 ounces baby spinach
- 3 tbsp soy sauce
- 1 tbsp sesame oil
- 1 stalk of shallots , sliced
- 1/4 cup pomegranate arils

Maple Dressing

- 1/4 cup + 1 tablespoons pure maple syrup
- 2 tablespoons Dijon Mustard
- 2 tablespoons White Balsamic Vinegar
- 1/4 cup mayo
- 3 tablespoons half & half
- Salt and pepper

Preparation:

1. Cook bulgur wheat. For that soak it in water overnight and boil until it softens for 15 minutes.
2. Slice butternut squash in half, take off the seeds. Preheat oven to 375 degrees F. Drizzle squash with olive oil and bake for 30 minutes.
3. Take the baked butternut squash and peel of the skin. Dice squash into medium cubes.
4. Mix all the Ingredients: including squash, spinach, seeds and bulgur.
5. Drizzle salad with Dijon dressing.
6. Serve hot.

Veggie Pizza

Ready in 40 minutes | Serves 1 person | 1030 calories

Ingredients:

- 2 mushrooms
- 30 grams of grated cheese
- 1 red bell pepper diced
- Ready pizza dough
- 1 zucchini
- 1 oz. olive oil or butter
- Salt and pepper
- Scallions
- Sun dried tomatoes in olive oil
- Tomato sauce

Preparation:

1. Spread your pizza dough in a round shape. Try to spread it as thin as possible for a better crust.
2. Dice zucchini into thin slices, bell pepper and mushrooms.
3. Spread tomato sauce over dough, try to cover as much as possible without gaps.
4. Put veggies on the pizza in the following order: zucchini first, then bell pepper and mushrooms, finish with sundried tomatoes and cheese evenly spread.
5. Preheat oven to 350 degrees F.
6. Spread oil or butter on a pizza pan. Place pizza in it.
7. Bake for 20-30 minutes.

Tips

Serve with fresh diced scallions, shaved parmesan or basil on top.

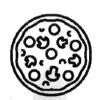

Tomato Basil Soup

Ready in 20 minutes | Serves 6 people | 280 calories per serving

Ingredients:

- 🍽 1 tablespoon olive oil
- 🍽 2 tablespoons butter
- 🍽 1 medium onion chopped
- 🍽 1 clove garlic minced
- 🍽 1 dash Italian seasoning
- 🍽 1 pack of chicken or veggie broth
- 🍽 1 can of whole or diced tomatoes peeled
- 🍽 Garlic croutons
- 🍽 Dried or fresh basil

Preparation:

1. Sauté onion in a soup pot until it's lightly browned;
2. Stir in the garlic, seasoning, tomatoes, and broth;
3. Simmer the soup for 8 minutes;
4. Blend the soup until smooth;
5. Stir in the cream, basil, add salt and pepper to taste, and serve

Tips

Serve with garlic croutons.

Thai Coconut Soup

Ready in 50 minutes | Serves 6 people | 312 calories

Ingredients:

- 2 Tbsp butter or coconut oil
- 1 yellow onion
- 4 Tbsp red Thai curry paste
- 1 lb. carrots
- 3 cuts of chicken or vegetable broth
- 1.3 oz. of coconut milk
- 4 stems of cilantro to taste for decoration
- 1 large sweet potato

Preparation:

1. In a large pan sauté the finely diced onion until soft and gold for about 5 minutes.
2. Once the onions are soft, add the Thai curry paste and continue to fry for about one mor minute.
3. While the onion is cooking, peel and dice the sweet potato into 1-inch cubes.
4. Add the sweet potato to the pot after the curry paste has sautéed, and let it simmer with sweet potatoes.
5. Peel and slice the carrots. Add the carrots to the pot thinly sliced.
6. Add vegetable broth to the pot, stir to combine, place a lid on top, and turn the heat up to high.
7. Allow the soup come to a boil, then turn the heat down to low (or just above low) and allow it to simmer for 30 minutes, stirring occasionally.
8. After 30 minutes the sweet potatoes and carrots should be extremely tender and fall apart as you stir the pot.

9. Turn the heat off and remove the pot from the hot stove top to facilitate cooling (to another area on the stove is fine). Add the coconut milk and stir to combine. You can reserve a tablespoon or two of the coconut milk to garnish the finished soup, if desired.

10. Put soup in a blender and process it to make a fine purée in.

11. Garnish with fresh cilantro and a bit of sriracha, to taste, salt and pepper.

Zucchini Fettuccine Pasta

Ready in 25 minutes | Serves 1 serving | 117 calories

Ingredients:

- 1 zucchini
- 1 oz. olive oil or butter
- Salt and pepper

Preparation:

1. Plan for roughly one medium-sized zucchini per person.
2. Split the zucchini in half lengthwise.
3. Scoop the seeds with a spoon and slice the halves very thinly with a potato peeler or use a spiralizer to make zucchini noodles .
4. Toss the zucchini noodles in a simmering water or tomato or cream sauce of your choice and serve immediately.
5. If you want to eat fewer calories, then parboil the zucchini slices for a minute and add olive oil or butter.
6. Salt and pepper to taste. Stir and serve.

Tips

Serve with fresh diced tomato, shaved parmesan and basil on top.

Butternut Squash Pasta with Pinenuts

Ready in 20 minutes | Serves 2 persons | 256 calories

Ingredients:

- ¼ cup of Pinenuts
- 1 butternut squash
- 1 oz. olive oil or butter
- ¼ cup of grated Parmesan
- Salt and pepper

Preparation:

1. Set oven to 350F. Chop up butternut squash, slicing horizontally into thick chunks, then peel or cut off the skin. Place future noodles on a baking sheet, spray with olive oil, then bake noodles for 6 to 8 minutes. Spray a skillet with olive oil, then add garlic and your choice of spice.
2. Once baked, slice into thin noodles.
3. Add oil or butter. Salt and pepper to taste.
4. Garnish with pinenuts and Parmesan. Stir and serve.

Tips

You can also serve with sundried tomatoes in oil, shaved parmesan and basil on top.

Fish Tacos

Ready in 10 minutes | Serves 1 person | 200 calories per taco

Ingredients:

- 1 pound tilapia fillets (a different variety of mild white fish will also work)
- 2 teaspoons olive oil
- 1 tablespoon taco seasoning
- 1 cup shredded cabbage
- 1 avocado (thinly sliced)
- 2 taco hard shells
- Fresh juice of 1 lime
- Salt and pepper

Preparation:

1. Marinade raw tilapia fillet in taco or Mexican seasoning and lime juice.
2. Take taco shell and fill it first with avocado, then cabbage, diced tilapia filet and finish with onion and diced tomatoes on top.
3. Add salt and pepper to taste.
4. Serve with a slice of lime.
5. Use sour cream or spicy salsa for sause.

Tips

Try to use fresh fish rather than frozen or canned.

Veggie Burrito

Ready in 20 minutes | Serves 1 person | 600 calories

Ingredients:

- 1/2 Medium Onion (Chopped)
- 1 Tbsp Olive Oil
- 1/4 tsp Cayenne Pepper
- 1/4 tsp Dried Chili Flakes
- 1/2 tsp Ground Cumin
- 1 large flour tortilla
- ½ cup of canned or cooked black beans
- 1 cup of shredded lettuce
- ½ cup of brown rice
- ½ cup of diced tomatoes
- ¼ cup of diced red onions
- ¼ cup of canned sweet corn
- 2 tbsp of sour cream
- 4 tbsp of hot salsa, optional

Preparation:

1. Mix rice with cumin, chili, cayenne spices add salt, ground pepper and oil.
2. Spread sour cream, and in the center of tortilla place beans, rice, lettuce, onions, corn and tomatoes, carefully leaving the edges empty so you can wrap it.
3. Wrap tortilla into a burrito and serve.

Tips

Serve with fresh diced tomato, shaved parmesan and basil on top.

Nachos with Guacamole Dip

Ready in 10 minutes | Serves 4 persons | 400 calories per serving

Ingredients:

- 4 cups of beef chili
- 4 large avocados
- 3/4 teaspoon salt
- juice from 2 small limes
- 4 cups frozen corn, thawed
- 1 pack of triangle nachos
- 50 grams of cheddar cheese
- 4 tbsp of sour cream

Preparation:

1. Place nachos onto a large plate. Put beef chili and cheese on top and microwave for 20 seconds, just until cheese melts.
2. Peel avocados. For that, slice them in half and take the seed out. Then take the inside with a spoon. Use ripe avocados only. Than process it in blender or smash it with a fork.
3. Put avocado sauce and sour cream on top and serve.
4. Serve hot.

Tips

For beef chilly saute 1 pound of minced beef with 1 can of blackbeans adding tex mex spices.

Try adding diced tomatoes, onions, corn and cilantro.

Veggie Panini

Ready in 15 minutes | Serves 1 person | 500 calories

Ingredients:

- 🍽 2 slices sourdough bread
- 🍽 light mayo
- 🍽 butter
- 🍽 1 slice colby jack cheese
- 🍽 6 leaves spinach
- 🍽 1 avocado
- 🍽 2 slices of tomato
- 🍽 1 small cucumber

Preparation:

1. Place veggies in layers with cheese on top on a slice of whole wheat bread covered with mayonnaise and cover with another slice of bread.
2. Put a panini sandwich on a press grill for 3 minutes and flip, hold for another 2 minutes.
3. Serve hot.

Chicken Caesar Wrap

Ready in 10 minutes | Serves 4 persons | 500 calories

Ingredients:

- 2 cups of cooked chicken, chopped
- 3 cups of Romaine lettuces, chopped
- 2/3 cup of cherry tomatoes , halved
- 1/4 cup of freshly grated parmesan cheese
- 4 flour tortilla wraps

For dressing:

- 1/2 cup croutons
- Juice of ½ lemon
- 4 tbsp of olive oil
- 2 cloves of garlic
- 4 tbsp of plain yogurt

Preparation:

1. Mix all the salad Ingredients: in a large bowl.
2. Dress salad with lemon juice, olive oil, yogurt and garlic mixture.
3. Put salad on a flour tortilla wrap, leaving the edges. Wrap and slice in half.
4. Put a toothpick through the halves to hold the wrap together.
5. Serve.

Caesar Salad with Salmon

Ready in 40 minutes | Serves 6 persons | 500 calories

Ingredients:

- 2 lbs salmon fillet, cut into 6 pieces
- Kosher salt
- Freshly ground black pepper
- 8 cups of Romaine lettuce
- ½ cup of Parmesan cheese
- 3 strips of fried bacon

Dressing Ingredients::

- 2 cloves garlic, minced
- 1 lemon
- 3 tbsp of olive oil
- Light mayonnaise or non-fat plain yogurt

Preparation:

1. Mix all the salad Ingredients: in a large bowl.
2. Dress salad with lemon juice, olive oil, yogurt and garlic mixture.
3. Grill or bake salmon fillets with salt and pepper and 1 tbsp of olive oil for 5-10 minutes.
4. Place salad on individual plates
5. Place ready salmon on top of a salad.
6. Serve with shavings of Parmesan cheese.

Tips

Try using shaved parmesan instead of processed one.

Chicken Donair Wrap

Ready in 4 hours | Serves 4 persons | 600 calories

Ingredients:

Marinade:

- 1/2 cup olive oil
- 1/4 cup lemon juice (from 2 lemons)
- 2 tsp smoked paprika
- 1/2 tsp tumeric
- 2 tsp cumin powder
- ⅓ cup mayonnaise
- ⅓ cup plain full fat yogurt
- 1 Large garlic clove, minced
- Salt and pepper to taste

For tsadziki sauce:

- ½ cup of Greek yogurt
- ½ cup of light mayonnaise
- 2 cloves of garlic
- ⅓ cup of shredded cucumber
- 4 Chicken skewers
- 1 Onion
- 2 tbsp of vinegar
- 4 pitas (or tortillas or lavash)
- 2 tomatoes
- 6 cups of lettuce, shredded
- 1 large cucumber, peeled and sliced
- 4 tbsp of hummus

Preparation:

1. Marinade chicken meat for 3-4 hours in a fridge. Mix all the Ingredients: and rub the chicken in it. Leave to rest.
2. Oven fry on broom setting chicken or BBQ it.
3. Prepare tsadziki sauce. Mix ⅓ cup of Greek yogurt, light mayonnaise with crushed garlic and ¼ cup of shredded cucumber.
4. On a pita or tortilla put hummus, tsadziki sause, lettuce, 4 half slices of tomato, marinated in vinegar onions, and grilled chicken kebab.
5. Serve hot.

Tips

Prepare marinade in the evening, so the chicken is marinated overnight.

Blue Cheese Pear Salad

Ready in 15 minutes | Serves 1 person | 380 calories

Ingredients:

- 2 generous handfuls leaves of your choice
- 2 pears, sliced
- 150g blue cheese, broken into chunks
- 50g crushed walnuts for sprinkling
- 60ml olive oil (4 Tbs)
- 1 boiled egg

Preparation:

1. Mix all the Ingredients: in a large bowl.
2. Dress with olive oil.
3. Place sliced boiled egg on top.

Kale Salad with Walnuts

Ready in 5 minutes | Serves 1 person | 280 calories

Ingredients:

- 4 large organic apples, sliced (or strawberries)
- 10 oz Kale Blend
- 1 cup raw walnuts
- 4 oz feta cheese, crumbled
- 1/3 cup dried cranberries
- 4 tbsp of olive oil

Preparation:

1. Mix all the Ingredients: in a large bowl.
2. Dress with olive oil.

Dinner

Dinner is the final meal of the day. It has to have all the nutrients, yet, not to be too heavy. You don't have to have only vegetables; it has to have protein. Treat yourself to meat chops, seafood and cheese, beans - those are the natural sources of protein that your body needs. Fish has necessary oils for beautiful skin and meat will ensure that you're building muscle after a hard day at gym or outside exercise. You can also treat yourself for a dessert.

Low-Carb Cajun Chicken

Ready in 45 minutes | Serves 4 person | 400 calories per serving

Ingredients:

- 2 teaspoons brown sugar substitute with agave syrup
- 1 1/2 teaspoons mild paprika
- 1 teaspoon dried oregano
- 1 teaspoon salt
- 1/2 teaspoon each garlic powder and onion powder
- 4 tbsp of olive oil
- 4 chicken brests

Preparation:

1. Mix all the spices in a small separate bowl.
2. Rub chicken breasts on both sides. Sprinkle with oil
3. Grease baking form with oil.
4. Place chicken breasts on baking form and bake for 25-35 minutes on high temperature.
5. Serve with a slice of lemon.

Stuffed Bell Peppers

Ready in 45minutes | Serves 6 person | 520 calories

Ingredients:

- 6 whole bell peppers (any color)
- 3/4 to 1 pound lean ground beef
- 1 white onion (diced)
- 3 cloves garlic (minced)
- 1 15 ounce can diced tomatoes, drained
- 1 cup cooked white rice
- 1 cup frozen corn
- 1 tablespoon Worcestershire sauce
- 1 1/2 teaspoon salt
- 1/2 teaspoon black pepper
- 1 1/2 cups shredded pepper jack cheese
- 250 ml of spicy tomato sauce

Preparation:

1. In a large bowl mix all the Ingredients: except for cheese and bell peppers.
2. Slice the tops of bell peppers and clear from seeds, making "cups" out of peppers.
3. Stuff peppers with a filling of rice, beef and veggies.
4. Bake for 40 minutes at 350 degrees F.
5. Take out of oven. Add grated cheese on top and bake for another 5 minutes.
6. Serve with spicy tomato sauce.

Stuffed Tomatoes

Ready in 8 minutes | Serves 1 person | 150 calories

Ingredients:

- 2 large tomatoes, preferably locally grown, washed
- 2 teaspoons extra virgin olive oil
- 1 teaspoon white wine vinegar, herb-infused vinegar preferable
- 2/3's cup cottage cheese
- 1/4 cup diced cucumber

Preparation:

1. Wash tomatoes and clear the inside from seeds. Slice the tops of tomatoes and take the inside with a spoon.
2. In a bowl mix cottage cheese, cucumber vinegar and oil.
3. Stuff tomatoes with cottage cheese.
4. Ready to serve.

Tips

Serve with a side of spinach salad or sweet potato mash.

Veggie Cabbage Rolls

Ready in 2 hours | Serves 6 persons | 300 calories

Ingredients:

- 10-12 Cabbage Leaves
- 1 Tablespoon (8.4 g) minced garlic
- 1 teaspoon (2.1 g) smoked paprika
- 2 teaspoons (1.6 g) thyme
- 2 pounds of cooked rice
- 1 can of tomato sauce
- 4 stems of celery
- Salt
- Ground pepper

Preparation:

1. Mix all the Ingredients: in a large bowl.
2. Boil cabbage head for 15-20 minutes.
3. Drain the water from cabbage.
4. Peel each cabbage leaf and please 2tbsp of filling in the middle. Roll the cabbage leaf up and stick the ends of the roll inside of it.
5. Do the same procedure with all the leaves until you run out of filling.
6. Place all the cabbage roll onto a casserole.
7. Cover with tomato sause or tomato juice and bake for 45 minutes at 350 degrees F.
8. Serve hot with sour cream.

Spicy Noodles with Chinese Mushrooms & Bach Choi

Ready in 25 minutes | Serves 4 persons | 200 calories

Ingredients:

- 1 Tablespoon oil
- 1 pound brown mushrooms sliced
- 5 ounces bamboo shoots drained, (1 short can)
- 1/2 pound baby bok choy stalks cut into quarters or eighths depending on size
- 2 green onions finely chopped
- 4 cloves garlic minced
- 1 Tablespoon ginger minced

Sauce

- 3 Tablespoons oyster sauce
- 2 Tablespoons of red wine or sherry
- 2 Tablespoons soy sauce
- 1/3 cup vegetable broth
- 2 teaspoons maple syrup
- 2 teaspoons cornstarch

Preparation:

1. Combine the Ingredients: for the sauce in a bowl. Mix well until fully combined.
2. Heat oil in a nonstick skillet over medium heat. Add ginger, garlic, and green onion. Stir for 2 minutes.
3. Add the mushrooms and stir for 2 minutes and bamboo shoots, stir for 3 minutes.
4. Add the baby bok choy, keep stirring, cover skillet, turn to low heat cook for 3 minutes.
5. Remove pan from heat. Shake or whisk the sauce with another stir to ensure the Ingredients: are well combined.
6. Pour the sauce into the skillet and stir well until it reaches even consistency.
7. Serve hot.

Spicy Thai Noodles

Ready in 30 minutes | Serves 4 persons | 192 calories

Ingredients:

- 1 9.5-ounce package udon noodles
- 2 tablespoons sesame oil
- 1 cup carrots, julienned
- 2 teaspoons fresh ginger, minced
- 1 cup shiitake mushrooms, sliced
- 4 green onions, sliced
- 4 tablespoons tamari
- 1 cup red bell peppers, julienned
- 1 teaspoon chili flakes (more if you like it spicy)
- 2 cloves garlic, minced
- 2 tablespoons honey
- 1 cup of cilantro, chopped
- 1/2 cup of Thai basil, chopped
- 1 tbsp of sesame seeds (optional)
- 1 lime wedges

Preparation:

1. Cook the udon noodles according to the directions on a package. Drain and set aside.
2. While the noodles are cooking, heat the sesame oil in a wok or large skillet over high heat.
3. Add the carrots, bell peppers and chili flakes and sauté for 2-3 minutes.
4. Add the garlic, ginger, mushrooms and green onions and stir fry for another 3 minutes.
5. In a small bowl, whisk together the tamari sauce and honey and add to the stir fried vegetables, stirring well.
6. Add the noodles and mix well. Cook just until noodles are heated through. Remove from heat and stir in the cilantro and basil.
7. Serve garnished with sesame seeds and lime wedges.

Tips

Serve Thai noodles while hot with a cucumber, mango salad or added tofu or chicken satay to add your favorite protein to this dish. Add a half-pound of uncooked cubed chicken, beef, tofu or satay shortly before you start to stir fry the vegetables.

Pesto Chicken Penne

Ready in 20 minutes | Serves 4 person | 400 calories

Ingredients:

- 2 pints cherry or grape tomatoes (about 4 cups)
- 1 tablespoon olive oil
- 1/2 teaspoon kosher salt, plus more for seasoning
- 1/4 teaspoon freshly ground black pepper, plus more for seasoning
- 4 boneless, skinless chicken breasts
- 100 g of Pesto sauce
- 1 pack of gluten free penne

Preparation:

1. Boil penne in a slightly salted water for 10-15 minutes.
2. Rub salt and pepper mix onto chicken breasts.
3. On a hot skillet pour oil and fry chicken until golden brown.
4. Slice chicken into strips and add to penne. Mix in pesto sauce.
5. Add sliced cherry tomatoes.

Tips

Serve with fresh diced tomato, shaved parmesan and basil on top.

Black bean Pasta with Sundried Tomato Pesto

Ready in 20 minutes | Serves 1 person | 200 calories

Ingredients:

- 1/2 onion finely chopped
- 100g sundried tomatoes in oil
- 150g mini portabella mushrooms
- A hand full of mixed deserved olives chopped up
- 400g tinned chopped tomatoes
- 200ml water
- 1/2 stock cube
- 1 heaped tsp of minced garlic
- 100g Black bean spaghetti
- 1 handful of basil leaves
- Black pepper

Preparation:

1. Fry mushrooms and onions adding oil, pepper, garlic.
2. Add water and stock cube, basil leaves and stir.
3. Boil black bean spaghetti al denté.
4. Add spaghetti to the sautés mushrooms, and stir fry for 3 minutes.
5. Add tinned tomatoes and let it simmer for 5 minutes.
6. Serve with sundried tomatoes and fresh basil.

Gluten-Free Pasta with Garlic Chicken

Ready in 30 minutes | Serves 4 person | 450 calories

Ingredients:

- 1 pound dried penne
- 2 chicken cutlets, cut into fingers
- Salt and freshly ground black pepper
- 3 cloves garlic, sliced
- 1/4 teaspoon red pepper flakes
- 3 tablespoons olive oil
- 3 tablespoons roughly chopped fresh parsley, for garnish
- 2 lemons, juiced
- 1/2 cup grated Parmesan

Preparation:

1. Cook the pasta in a large pot of boiling salted water, until al dente. Drain well.
2. Season chicken with salt and pepper. Heat a large grill pan over medium high and add chicken. Grill until golden and completely cooked. Remove to a plate and slice.
3. Add the garlic and red pepper flakes to a saute pan with 3 tablespoons of olive oil and saute until fragrant. Add the cooked pasta and turn heat off. Mix all together.
4. Remove pasta to a large bowl. Add chicken to the warm pasta and season with salt and pepper. Sprinkle in chopped parsley. Add the juice of 2 lemons and mix. Serve warm.

Tips

Serve with fresh shaved parmesan and basil on top.

Gluten-Free Pasta with Seafood

Ready in 20 minutes | Serves 4 persons | 300 calories

Ingredients:

- 4 Tbsp butter, divided
- 8 oz seafood mix
- 4 cloves garlic
- 28 oz can whole peeled tomatoes
- 1 cup of spicy tomato sauce
- 1/4 tsp red pepper flakes (optional)
- 1 pack of gluten-free linguine
- Fresh basil for garnish

Preparation:

1. On a hot skillet put butter. Add garlic and fry for two minutes. Then add finely diced tomatoes. Add pepper flakes.
2. Add seafood mix to garlic and fry for another 8-15 minutes.
3. Separately boil linguine to al denté. Add to the seafood.
4. Add tomato sauce and let it simmer for another 5 minutes.

Tips

Serve with a slice of lemon and basil on top.

Grilled Cod with Asparagus and Béchamel Sauce

Ready in 50 minutes | Serves 1 person | 350 calories

Ingredients:

- asparagus spears (ends trimmed) 1 lbs 454 g
- cod filets (4-ounce each, rinsed and patted dry)
- 2 tbsp of olive oil

For sauce Béchamel:

- 3 egg yolks
- 1 stick of butter
- fresh lemon juice
- salt
- pepper

Preparation:

1. Grill or fry cod fillet for five minutes. Do not overlook it as the meat will become rubbery because of high protein content.
2. Add salt and pepper. Do not put salt before cooking fish. Fillet will release water and will not be juicy.
3. Fry asparagus for 10-15 minutes on olive oil.
4. Prepare Béchamel sauce. For Béchamel sauce whisk egg yolks, 1/4 cup water and 2 Tbsp. fresh lemon juice in small saucepan until blended.
5. Cook over very low heat, stirring constantly, until mixture bubbles at the edges.
6. Stir in butter, one piece at a time, until butter is melted and until sauce is thickened.
7. Remove from heat.
8. Stir in spices.
9. It should make about ¾ of a cup of sauce.
10. On a large plate place asparagus first and cod on top. Pour sauce over. Serve warm while sauce is still hot.

Tips

Serve with a slice of lemon.

Beef Chop with Sweet Potato Mash

Ready in 45 minutes | Serves 4 persons | 500 calories

Ingredients:

- 2 tablespoons salt-reduced soy sauce
- 2 tablespoons mirin (rice wine)
- 1 teaspoon honey
- 4 (about 125g each) beef fillet steaks
- 700g orange sweet potato (kumara), peeled, coarsely chopped
- 4 tbsp of olive oil
- 2 teaspoons finely grated ginger
- 1 long fresh red chili, deseeded, finely chopped
- 1 tablespoon chopped fresh coriander
- Steamed Asian greens, to serve

Preparation:

1. Bake sweet potatoes at high heat for 20 minutes.
2. Remove from the oven and peel.
3. Mash potatoes and add olive oil to it, salt and pepper.
4. Take the meat chop and rub salt and pepper in it.
5. Mix honey, rice vinegar, chili and olive oil.
6. Fry your chop on a hot skillet adding honey mix.
7. Serve hot with sweet potato mash on a side.

Ginger Beef with Steamed Vegetables

Ready in 20 minutes | Serves 2 persons | 300 calories

Ingredients:

- 1 lb. skirt steak, thinly sliced into ¼ inch strips
- kosher salt
- Freshly ground black pepper
- 1 tsp. plus 1 tbsp. olive oil
- 1 lb. green beans, trimmed
- 3 cloves garlic, minced
- 3 inch piece of ginger, peeled and finely grated
- 1/4 cup of light soy sauce or may use more concentrated one for zest
- 1 tbsp. rice wine vinegar
- 3 tbsp. sugar
- 2 green onions, chopped
- 1 tbsp. sesame seeds

Preparation:

1. Place beef in a large mixing bowl and pat dry with paper towels. Season with salt and pepper, toss and set aside.
2. In a large skillet over medium-high heat, pour 1 tbsp of olive oil and cook beans for 1 minute. Add 2 tbsp of water and cover with a lid to steam and cook for two more minutes.
3. Transfer green beans to a plate and discard any excess water.
4. Return pan to high heat and drizzle it with remaining tablespoon of oil. When oil is hot, add beef. Stir-fry until beef is cooked through for 3 to 5 minutes.
5. Reduce to medium heat and add garlic, soy sauce, vinegar, and sugar and ginger, stir quickly to coat the beef. Add back green beans, and top with diced green onions and sesame seeds.

Tips

Serve warm and fresh.

Lamb Shashlyk

Ready in 4 hours | Serves 4 persons | 250 calories

Ingredients:

- 1 large onion, peeled and finely grated
- 1 tablespoon lemon juice, strained if fresh
- 1 tablespoon olive oil
- 1 teaspoon salt
- ¼ teaspoon black pepper, freshly ground
- 2 lbs boneless lamb shoulder or 2 lbs leg of lamb, cut into 1 inch cubes
- 2 medium onions, cut into 1/4 inch chunks

Preparation:

1. Cut lamb into 2-inch chunks.
2. Prepare marinade with oil, onion, salt, pepper and lemon juice.
3. Marinade shashlyk for at least 2 hours under press.
4. Cut onions into rings and put chunk of meat and an onion ring on a skewer, interchangeably. Put about 4 pieces of meat and 4 onion rings per skewer.
5. Grill for 15 to 20 minutes.

Tips

Serve with lemon.

Tuna Ceviche

Ready in 20 minutes | Serves 1 person | 250 calories

Ingredients:

- 1 pound of sushi grade tuna cut in ¼ inch dice (or shrimp)
- 1/4 cup red onion diced
- 1-2 serrano or jalapeno peppers seeded and finely diced
- 1 ripe avocado diced
- 1/4 cup extra virgin olive oil

Preparation:

1. In a bowl mix the ingredients.
2. Season with oils.
3. Make sure all of Ingredients are finely diced.
4. Servewith nachos or pita chips

Desserts

Treat yourself to a dessert when hit a desired weight target. Keto diet is not only healthy, but also tasty. Low calorie desserts and snacks are perfect for a sweet tooth who does not want to give up habit of having desserts.

Oatmeal Cookies

Ready in 55 minutes | Serves 32 cookies | 421 calories

Ingredients:

- 1 1/2 cups of all-purpose flour, leveled
- 1 tsp ground cinnamon
- 1/2 tsp baking soda
- 1/2 tsp baking powder
- 1/2 tsp salt
- 4 eggs
- 1 cup of sugar
- ½ cup of brown sugar
- 2 cups of oats
- ½ cup of raisins
- ½ cup of butter or 1 stick
- 1 tsp of vanilla extract

Preparation:

1. Beat four eggs. Add white sugar and brown sugar, vanilla extract and cinnamon, salt and soda.
2. Melt butter.
3. Add melted butter and blend well.
4. Add flour, baking powder and oats. Mix well. Add raisins.
5. Mix all the Ingredients:.
6. Grease a baking form with butter or oil.
7. Form small balls of 3 cm in diameter and place them on a baking form with an interval of 3 cm.
8. Preheat oven to 280 degrees F.
9. Bake for 8 minutes.
10. Take from the oven, cover with a clean kitchen towel and let it cool for 15 minutes.
11. Serve warm while it's chewy.

Angelfood Cake with Raspberry Sauce

Ready in 55 minutes | Serves 10 persons | 257 calories per 100 grams

Ingredients:

- 1 and 3/4 cups (350g) granulated sugar
- 1 cup and 2 Tablespoons (130g) of cake flour
- 1/4 teaspoon of Kosher salt
- 12 large egg whites
- 1 and 1/2 teaspoons cream of tartar
- 2 tbsp of icing sugar to decorate
- ½ lemon
- 4 cups of fresh raspberries

Preparation:

1. Beat egg whites with pinch of salt. Gradually add sugar while whipping . Beat up egg whites until it forms a thick firm foam. Whip for 15-20 minutes.
2. Add cream of tartar and beat for another minute.
3. Gradually add sifted flour while whipping.
4. Spread oil or butter onto the baking form, make sure to get sides oiled so the cake does not stick to it.
5. Pour cake batter into a baking form and bake in preheated oven for 30 minutes at 350 degrees F.
6. Take the cake out of the oven and let it cool off for 20 minutes.
7. Take it out of the baking form by flipping it upside down.
8. Decorate with icing sugar and raspberries.
9. Serve with raspberry sauce or jam.
10. For raspberry sauce take 1 cup of fresh raspberries and ¼ cup of sugar and process it in blender. Add juice of half a lemon. Pour sauce over a slice of cake and serve.

Chocolate Mousse

Ready in 1 hour 20 minutes | Serves 4 persons | 225 calories per 100 grams

Ingredients:

- 4 large egg yolks
- 1/4 cup sugar
- 2 1/2 cups heavy whipping cream
- 8 oz semisweet baking chocolate, chopped

Preparation:

1. Place chocolate in a large bowl set over a bain marie or in a double boiler at a low simmer. Stir chocolate until melted. Turn off the heat and let stand.
2. Beat the cream over ice until it forms soft peaks. Set aside and hold at room temperature. With a mixer, whip egg to soft peaks. Gradually add the sugar and continue whipping until firm.
3. Remove the chocolate from the bain marie and using a whisk, fold in the egg whites all at once.
4. When the whites are almost completely incorporated, fold in the whipped cream.
5. Cover the mousse and refrigerate for approximately 1 hour or until set.
6. Serve in goblets topped with more whipped cream and shaved chocolate, if desired.

Low-Calorie Vanilla Custard

Ready in 40 minutes | Serves 1 person | 214 calories

Ingredients:

- 1 vanilla pod
- 2 ½ cup of 2% milk
- 4 large organic egg yolks
- 2 tablespoons sugar or brown sugar or syrup
- 1 tablespoon of cornflour

Preparation:

1. Onto a pan on a medium-low heat, pour in the milk and bring just to the boil. Add scraped out seeds of vanilla and the pod itself.
2. Remove from the heat and leave to chill slightly, then take out the vanilla pod.
3. In a large mixing bowl, whisk the egg yolks with sugar and cornflour until they form a foam.
4. Gradually add the warm milk, a small amount at a time, whisking well before each addition.
5. Pour the mixture back into the pan and cook gently on a low heat for about 20 minutes until thickened, stirring continuously.

Tips

Served better with a fruit crumble.

Avocado Truffles

Ready in 10 minutes | Serves 1 person | 92 calories per 1 truffle

Ingredients:

- 6 oz. of dark chocolate
- 1/3 cup mashed avocado (about 1 small avocado)
- 1/2 teaspoon vanilla extract
- pinch of salt
- 2 tablespoons cocoa powder, for rolling (optional)

Preparation:

1. Melt chocolate. Use a pot and a bowl. Put boiling water in one, place a metal bowl on top of it with chocolate chunks.
2. Mix all the ingredients: including melted chocolate.
3. Form even balls with 1-inch diameter.
4. Roll balls in cocoa powder to make them less sticky and to decorate them.

Mango Pudding

Ready in 2 hours | Serves 4 persons | 167 calories

Ingredients:

- 3 middle size mature mangoes (fresh mango cubes 1 pound)
- 2 packet unflavored gelatin sheets (or 10g, see the pack for instructions if you want to use gelatin powder)
- 160 ml milk or coconut milk
- 60 ml heavy cream, chilled
- 1/2 cup granulated sugar

Preparation:

1. Peel mangoes and make a pure by processing it in blender.
2. Boil 1 cup of water and dissolve gélatine sheets in it.
3. Add mango pure to it along with coconut milk and heavy cream m.
4. Mix well and let it chill for few hours.
5. Serve when mango pudding is set solid and "shaky" when touched.

Tips

Serve with slices of fresh fruit and whipped cream.

Stuffed Apples

Ready in 30 minutes | Serves 4 persons | 300 calories

Ingredients:

- 4 golden apples
- 2 cups of cream cheese
- ½ cup of raisins
- 1 tsp of vanilla extract
- 1 tbsp of honey or brown sugar
- ¼ cup of crushed walnuts

Preparation:

1. Wash apples. Slice the tops and hollow out the inside with seeds. The hole must be about an inch.
2. Mix walnuts, raisins and cream cheese. Add vanilla extract and mix.
3. Put honey or brown sugar on the bottom of each apple.
4. Stuff apples with cream cheese.
5. Bake for 15-20 minutes at low heat. Check on apples after 15 minutes.
6. Serve hot.

Tips

Serve with honey on top.

Coconut Bombs

Ready in 20 minutes | Serves 10 bombs | 302 calories

Ingredients:

- 3 oz. unsalted butter
- 1/2 cup unsweetened shredded coconut
- 1/4 tsp ground cardamom (green)
- 1/2 tsp vanilla extract
- 1/4 tsp ground cinnamon

Preparation:

1. Mix well all the Ingredients: and roll into balls to form a perfect coconut bomb.
2. Let it set. You may also bake it for 5 minutes until golden brown for a crunch.
3. Serve.

Planning Your Meal

To start loosing weight effectively you have to keep on track and eat well, avoiding occasional fast food snacks and handy premade processed foods. It is hard to stay focused on a diet with a modern pace of life, in this case planning your meal will help you and make it much more east. Make a grocery list and cook a week full of food on weekends. Stack up your fridge with healthy homemade meals in zip lock containers and will not have to worry. Moreover, most of the meals do not take more than 20 minutes to make, so you can live a healthy lifestyle without putting extra time into it, just living at a usual normal pace, but eating healthy.

Diet Recommendations

To ensure your body is healthy and metabolizes well, it is important to make meal intakes systematic i.e. at the same certain time. To make sure that body got used to diet and it is easier for you to switch, do not make your diet shorter than 21 day. In 3 week, period you will get used to new foods and new more active lifestyle and hence, will do your exercises with pleasure and will not think as much of unhealthy food options.

Before starting Keto diet it is highly advised to check with your doctor or talk to a professional dietician specialist if you have concerns or health related issues.

How to Lose Weight in 21 Days

To lose weight effectively and fast reprogram your thinking. 21-day program will let you do it step by step and will give you enough time to accommodate diet to your busy lifestyle. The variety of food recipes suggested will give you plenty of options to mix and create your own Keto diet meal plan. Combine Keto diet with after gym protein shakes. Replace regular sugars with healthier agave syrup, honey or brown sugar. Eat less but more frequently. Eat more colorful foods, greens, vegetables, replace starchy products with salads. Eat whole wheat instead of white bread. Replace heavy meals with light snacks, salads and wraps. Soups will help you to detox. Eat lots of celery and roots. Replace regular animal protein with vegetable protein like chickpeas, black and white kidney beans, eat more fish.

21 Day Meal Plan

Day 1

Breakfast: Eggs Benedict (See page 31)

Lunch: Italian Wedding Soup | Stuffed Bell Peppers (See page 65)

Dinner: Garlic Chicken Breast and Zucchini (See page 73)

Snack: Coconut Trail Mix

Day 2

Breakfast: Egg Salad (See page 33)

Lunch: Tomato Basil Soup (See page 48)

Dinner: Pasta with Seafood (See page 74)

Snack: Chocolate Mousse (See page 84)

Day 3

Breakfast: Scrambled Eggs and Bacon (See page 13)

Lunch: Stuffed Tomatoes (See page 66)

Dinner: Butter Chicken with Rice

Snack: Nutrition Bar

Day 4

Breakfast: Deviled Eggs

Lunch: Kale Salad with Walnuts (See page 62)

Dinner: Pesto Chicken with Steamed Veggies (See page 71)

Snack: Banana Chocolate Smoothie (See page 42)

Day 5

Breakfast: Breakfast Burrito

Lunch: Shwarma wrap

Dinner: Ginger Beef with Rice (See page 78)

Snack: Pomegranate Smoothie (See page 37)

Day 6

Breakfast: Breakfast Burrito

Lunch: Salmon with Quinoa

Dinner: Tikka Masala

Snack: Mango Smoothie (See page 39)

Day 7

Breakfast: Feta Cheese Wrap (See page 29)

Lunch: Blackbean Pasta with Red Pesto

Dinner: Cauliflower Fritters and Ranch Salad (See page 15)

Snack: Chia Pudding (See page 41)

Day 8

Breakfast: Chicken Fritters

Lunch: Butternut Squash with Bulgur Bowl (See page 46)

Dinner: Cod Fish with Asparagus under sauce Béchamel (See page 75)

Snack: Coffee with Biscotti

Day 9

Breakfast: Apple Pancakes (See page 20)

Lunch: Pear and Blue Cheese Salad (See page 61)

Dinner: Fish Tacos (See page 53)

Snack: Celery Veggie Smoothie

Day 10

Breakfast: Banana Waffles (See page 22)

Lunch: Tofu Udon and Veggie Curry

Dinner: Sushi

Snack: A Slice of Pumpkin Pie

Day 11

Breakfast: Strawberry Banana Pancakes (See page 21)

Lunch: Carrot Soup and a Whole Wheat Turkey Panini

Dinner: Ceviche

Snack: Vanilla Custard (See page 22)

Day 12

Breakfast: Breakfast Cereal with Coconut

Lunch: Chicken Caesar Salad Wrap (See page 57)

Dinner: Korean Style Spring Rolls with Glass Noodles

Snack: Mango Pudding (See page 87)

Day 13

Breakfast: 2 Small Oatmeal Muffins

Lunch: Spicy Thai Soup or Roasted fennel and snow pea salad

Dinner: Wok with Bach Choi and Chinese Mushrooms

Snack: Ginger Smoothie (See page 38)

Day 14

Breakfast: Eggs and Turkey Sausage

Lunch: Seafood Noodle Bowl

Dinner: Garlic Chicken (See page 73)

Snack: Greek Yougurt

Day 15

Breakfast: Breakfast Cereal with Chocolate Chips (See page 25)

Lunch: Stuffed Mushrooms

Dinner: Chicken Cutlets with Greens

Snack: Macaroons

Day 16

Breakfast: Poached Eggs and Avocado Sandwich (See page 28)

Lunch: Spicy Fish with Rice

Dinner: Polish Casserole with Sauerkraut

Snack: Low-calorie Raspberry jam

Day 17

Breakfast: Cottage Cheese Stuffed Apples (See page 88)

Lunch: Greek Salad and Yougurt

Dinner: Beef Tartar

Snack: Chickpea Hummus Dip with Pita Chips

Day 18

Breakfast: Breakfast Cereal with Berries

Lunch: French Onion Soup with Garlic Croutons

Dinner: Butternut Squash Pasta with Bulgur
and Pinenuts (See page 52)

Snack: Avocado Truffles

Day 19

Breakfast: Orange Smoothie

Lunch: Vegan Cabbage Rolls with Tomato Sauce (See page 67)

Dinner: Pork Chop with Sweet Potato Mash

Snack: Mango Pudding (See page 87)

Day 20

Breakfast: Breakfast Fajita

Lunch: Zucchini Pasta (See page 51)

Dinner: Lamb Shashlyk with Green Bell Peppers (See page 79)

Snack: Coconut Bombs (See page 89)

Day 21

Breakfast: Mango Smoothie (See page 87)

Lunch: Green Peas Soup with Croutons

Dinner: Low Carb Cajun Chicken (See page 64)

Snack: Nachos with Guacamole Dip (See page 55)

Disclaimer

This book contains opinions and ideas of the author and is meant to teach the reader in an informative way the information provided. The instructions may not be suitable for everyone. Using this book and implementing the information/recipes, therein, contained is explicitly your own responsibility and risk. This work with all its contents, does not guarantee completion or correctness of the provided information.

Design: Oliviaprodesign

Picture: **YARUNIV Studio** / www.shutterstock.com

Printed in Great Britain
by Amazon

40606615R00066